STOP DIABETES
in IT'S TRACKS..."GONE"

DAVIT LAMBERT SR.

ISBN 979-8-9874106-0-8

HEALTH = WEALTH

Health = Wealth

Contributors : resource

Centers for Disease Control and Prevention information factors [CDC].

Food and Drug Administration [FDA] rules and regulations.

Health and Human Service the Department for Sister Agencies (CDC and FDA)

Public Library of Science (PLOS)

World Health Organization (WHO)

International Agency for Research on Cancer (IARC)

TAKE YOUR LIFE BACK
NO MORE : DIABETES

Statistic /Study of the Diabetes Exposure! CDC: OF US ADULTS HAVE DIABETES, WITH FEWER NEW CASES

Approximately 34.1 million U.S. adults-more than 1 in 10-have type one or type 2 diabetes, and 7.3 million of those adults who met laboratory criteria were unaware or did not report having the disease, according to data from the CDC`s 2020 National Diabetes Statistics Report.

34.2 million Americans- just over 1 in 10-have diabetes. 88 million american adults-Approximately 1 in 3 have pre diabetes. New diabetes cases were higher among Non-Hispanics Orgin than Non-Hispanics Asians and Non-Whites.

SEPT. 2018

FEB. 11,2020

NATIONAL DIABETES STATISTIC REPORT,/2020 CDC

And statistic on diabetes and it`s burden in the United States Formerly know... however, as type 2 diabetes accounts for 90% to 95% of all diabetes cases. The data presented here are more likely... RISK FACTOR ABCs Goals for many adults.

FEB. 25,2020

CDC: 13% of U.S. Adults have diabetes with fewer new cases. The total direct and indirect costs of diagnosed in the U.S. was estimated at $327 billion for 2017. Between 2012 and 2017, excess medical costs per person associated with diabetes increased from $8,417 to $9,601 (2017 dollars). 1.5 Million diagnose every year. 100 Million adults living with diabetes or pre diabetes by Center for control.

CDC: SEPT. 22, 2018 14% of U.S. adults have diabetes many unaware of the disease status. Type 2 diabetes can progress over extended times.

NICHOLAS D. MENDOLA a student volunteer with the national center for Health Statistics (NCHS)" WROTE DATA BRIEF") " If left unmanaged, diabetes my contribute to serious health outcomes including Neuropathy ,Nephropathy , Retinopathy, Coronary Artery disease, Stroke and Peripheral Vascular disease". Additionally, total diabetes prevalence was higher among all minority groups; prevalence was highest among Hispanic adults (19.8%) followed by black adults (17%) and Asian Adults (15.3%) vs White adults (12.4%). Researcher also found diabetes prevalence increased with increase weight status category from 6.2% among adults with Underweight or Normal weight, to 11.8% among adults with Overweight to 20.7% among adults with Obesity.

Among children and adolescents, overall incidence of type 1 diabetes increased between 2002 and 2015 with largest increase observed among HiSpanic children.

Between 2002 and 2015, overall incidence <u>type 2 diabetes among children and adolescents also increased</u>, with changes consistent across racial groups.

Parents with all of our help, let`s go all out! to change our ways, to change the intake diet of sugar for all childred in the WORLD. *DEL*

METFORMIN CANCER HISTORY

On Dec. 5, 2019, the FDA issued a statement that was investigating the possible presence of NDMA (known as N-Nitrosodimethylamine) in metformin. At the time, the FDA said that some international regulatory agencies announced a metformin recall, but it would test the diabetes medication for high levels of the carcinogen.

NDMA has an acceptable daily intake limit 96 nanograms. It is classified as probably carcinogenic to humans by the World Health Organization (WHO) and the International Agency for Research on Cancer (IARC).

On March 2 2020, online pharmacy Valisure announced it tested 38 batches of metformin from 22 companies and found 16 batches from 11 companies with unacceptably high NDMA levels. Some batches contain more than 10 times the daily acceptable NDMA limits.

Valisure then filed a Citizen Petition with FDA, requesting the agency issue a recall of metformin products containing dangerous NDMA levels. The pharmacy also requested enhanced metformin NDMA testing. "On

June 11, 2020, the FDA announced it found high levels of NDMA in extended-release metformin HCL 500 mg made by five companies."

- Apotex Inc- All lots
- Amneal Pharmaceuticals LLC- All lots
- Marksans Pharma LTD (labeled as Time-Cap) - One lot (xp9004)
- Lupin Ltd-One lot (G901203)
- Teva Pharmaceuticals (labeled as Activist)-14 lots

The more side effect of metformin include: Heartburn, stomach pain, nausea or vomiting, bloating, gas, diarrhea, constipation, weight loss. Metformin Side Effects-Health line: physical weakness (asthenia), diarrhea, gas(flatulence),symptoms of weakness, muscle pain in (myalgia) ,upper respiratory tract infection, low blood sugar (hypoglycemia),abdominal pain (GI complaints), lactic acidosis (rare),low blood levels of vitamin.

PLOS ONE: stated under methods: We conducted the Systematic According to the Preferred Reporting items for Systematic Reviews and Meta-Analyses (Prism) Statement and Cochrane Collaboration guidelines [18] (Table S1) we searched Medline and Embrace (January 1966 to April 2012) for Randomized and Observational studies of the association between metformin and cancer in patient with diabetes mellitus.

STUDY SELECTION : We selected the following study designs :a) Prospective , Randomized, controlled, open or blinded traits (RCTs) enrolling patients with diabetes mellitus than one publication of one study Allocated to Metformin Treatment or a control group (Active Control or Placebo : b) cohort studies, case control or nested case control studies of patients with diabetes mellitus that reported data on exposure to metformin therapy and cancer incidence (Prevalence or Cancer mortality :c) studies in which exposure to metformin was assessed from prescription database, and incidence of cancer was derived from cancer registries. Where more than one publication of one study existed, we used the most complete database Recent Publication.

THAT BIG BAD WORD !
DIABETES...Stop"
DIABETS" IN IT`s TRACKS,WITH NO MEDICEN BUT WITH WHAT GOD HAS ALREADY GIVEN US.

I had been TYPE 2 for years: I got my first unannounced appearance in the 90`s, when I had to pack a gallon of water up stairs every night until, I could get to my Doctors appointment.

When I got to the Doctors office, he said, I have DIABETES. He told me I could be put on INSULIN or take a pill, of course I chose the pill. I had watch my mother give herself the shot and I told myself, I would never have to do that, I was 21yrs old at the time.

My Doctor started me on MEDAFORMIN. I was on it for quite a will. Then one day I got some information that it was not good for you, and I stopped taking it.

One day I was driving down the road and start shacking , SLOWLY THEN IT GOT WORSE. Instantly I took myself to the hospital. They finally checked me in and diagnose my glucose was extremely high. They got it under control and admitted me in.

I remained there for about a week. Then they put me on 50mg of insulin a day and released me. After about a year I got it down to about 40mg a day. Doing everything according to the book and following my dietitian and all the dietetics information.

I started Exercising (E) and eating the correct Foods (F), and as it improved , I started adjusting the amount of INSULIN, and keep my Doctors informed on my next visit.

The correct foods I used, I will announce later. I suggest you have to have FAITH, it will not happen overnight. But you will began to feel better all the time. When I was in the hospital a Doctor stated to me with a smirk laugh! You will have to take the insulin for LIFE. That was a shock to me, already nerves and too see and here with a laugh forever . I let myself believe it.

Then though about my cousin, She told me she had gotten redd of her diabetes by taken cinnamon and exercising per her doctor. She was not on insulin. She was a Type 1.

My doctors, was always trying to put me on insulin, but I refuse to use the needle. They were aware that metformin was not good. I told myself! I would never get on the needle, but when you are faced with a no choice situation you will say ok or yes. All of my words I had to eat, I was now on the needle.

To make a long story short , I started going to the GYM, why I had not prior? I don`t know when my insurance was telling me it was covered. When I started! it felt good. When I was in high school I played football, ran track, basketball, and swimming. In college I took weight lifting classes for PE.

It takes discipline and hard work but to get your life back together in this life time, it is so easy and how great of a reward for you. There`s lots of medicine, out there that supposed to help you, if you continue to use it. "WOW" all have great side effects, you may die from some of the side effects! Who wants that scare?

You will have to all ways , check your GLUCOSE every day. I check mine every morning and every night at the same time. Once you get off of insulin and/or medicine. WHY? Because your glucose: it can get to low and/or to high and that can help you stay health by correcting your food intake. Whatever the numbers are, don`t panic just wait and correct your intake. It will be a balancing act but you will always know what your numbers are.

Best thing to remember is don`t panic. A high doesn`t mean you got to take a shot or medicine. What it does say" OH" I get to get it under control. With proper eating and exercise.

Do the right thing for eating. Don`t eat late and eat lighter at night and eat a heavy breakfast. Drink lots of water, it flushes out sugar. So if you go to the rest room at night more you are removing sugar. No sugar drinks, it goes straight to your stomach, normally the size of your stomach is the problem.

People say sugar has not anything to do with diabetes. I say sugar is like POSION. Our parents gave it to use because their parents did the same, when they were a child. The food system is set up to keep you HOOKED On, taste to get you to come back. There`s lots of hidden sugar SO YOU OWE IT TO

YOURSELF. TO investigate everything you put in your mouth. Number one thing to remember, ask GOD through prayer to help you. Too get Healing from the DIVINE.

There is not an evil thing in eating or drinking something you are craving for, but which one is most important to you! Self -fulfillment (gratification) or your health. Do everything in moderation.

I did not get off the needle all at once. When I started eating and exercising properly. I was able to reduce the insulin according to the readings I was getting doing my testing. When I left the hospital I was taking 50mg per day, 25mg in the morning and 25mg at night.

As I start losing weight! Oh yes you will lose weight. The most important part of your body is to help control your stomach size.

You have to take this thing seriously. I have no medical studies. I have an Aeronautics Engineer degree.

Doing my reduction of insulin, on my visit to the doctor, I informed them of my reduction. I was taking 10mg in the morning and 10mg at night. FEB. 2020, I was on a trip in Houston and realized I left my insulin at home .Called and had it shipped. The next morning, I checked my blood glucose monitor and my level was about the same, as if I had taken it the night before. I said 'WOW' how`s that possible. That night before eating I checked it and the numbers was good as if I had taken insulin. The package arrived the next day. I didn`t open it.

I told all of my Doctors they said keep monitoring it. So continue to get your blood checked by your doctor. And learn to experiment with your dosages until you know you have t under control. Always monitor your glucose. If your sugar goes to low make sure you keep some hard candy or peanut butter nearby . If it gets to high just control your food intake until you get it under control. One of my doctors you got it under control.

I recently received information from my KIDNEY DR. He said my kidney numbers was good, and my blood count was better, improved anemic.

FOOD:

I suggest to eating raw vegetables and find out what vegs works good for you, by your readings (checks). I eat no RED MEATS, no PROCESS foods. I eat Fish_and Chicken_but more Fish. I eat SUGAR free Bread. When I am eating the RAW VEGS., I use an Extra Virgin Olive OIL and drizzle a Sugar Free SYRUP on top as a sweet taste and include raw strawberries and blue berries. Also green peppers, red pepper, yellow pepper, orange peppers, spinach and red onion as my salad. (I CAN`T WAIT TO EAT THE SALAD) it is so good. For breakfast I eat Oatmeal .

What is so good about the sugar free bread is I use it as a snack . Also one important snack I eat chocolate 90% COCOA for your heart as a snack, only eat a small amount per day. Also I eat sugar free gel snack (Jello) . Eat everything in moderation , don`t over eat anything.. Always eat three meals per day. Heavy in the morning and lighter at night.

THE SECRET FORMAL FOR HEALTH

GOD [or whom you believe in]

DIABETES   FOODS

EXERSISE

DIABETS + GOD +FOODS   = LIFE HEALTH
EXERCISE

©

Today due to COV-19 I don`t go to the GYM. I use the parks and my garage to exercise. You should at least exercise 20 min. a day or longer.

There is something that is EXTRAORDINARY about this special formula beside getting off the needle(INSULANT) . That is! the medicine I am able to get ride of. I was taking three (3) different medications for my blood pressure a day , now I am only taking one(1) . I was taking meds. for acid reflux , I no longer take anything for it, (**Gone**).

18 years and over	209,128,094	74.3
Male	100,994,367	35.9
Female	108,133,727	38.4
21 years and over	196,899,193	70.
Total	615,155,381	

13% 79,970,199.53

2017) 1.5 million diagnosed every year

100 million living with diabetes or pre diabetes

Davit Lambert author of STOP Diabetes in its TRACKS...Gone.

Davit Lambert lives in Dallas,TX. Has a Aeronautical Engineering Degree. Davit has a Mobile machine service. Has been racing automobiles since age 15. Davit has 25 years of experience in the Corporate Restaurant Management industry. Davit love sports, Football, Basketball, ect..

Ingram Content Group UK Ltd.
Milton Keynes UK
UKHW050638190423
419951UK00038B/152

9 798987 410608